Foods for Your Brain & Emotions

Foods for Your Brain & Emotions

Food Wisdom Series

By Miriam Moras

Foods for Your Brain & Emotions

About Broccoli People

Broccoli People's books aim to provide accessible and practical information on health and nutrition. In today's world, the amount of information and controversies can be confusing and overwhelming. Therefore, the objective here is to simplify these topics.

The author, Miriam Moras, a health coach specialised in nutrition, created this series with the intention to offer simple and accessible guides emphasising the holistic nature of health and well-being.

You won't find the latest trendy diets or new products, but rather guidelines to be adapted for each person. However, the fields of nutrition and well-being are constantly evolving, and there is always much left to be discovered. As a result, there have already been several revisions to keep the books up-to-date.

Afterward, if you are interested and want to explore specific topics further, you can continue your journey of learning and exploring life as a never ending process.

As Marie Curie said,

"Nothing is to be feared, only to be understood."

"Foods for Your Brain & Emotions"

There is much we don't understand about the brain yet, but we know that it plays a crucial role in our quality of life, and that our daily choices can also impact its well-being. Our emotions, ability to deal with life's challenges, concentration, and mental thriving are all affected by our physical health, particularly the brain and neurological system.

The body and brain can be compared to machines, and the food we consume is like the fuel they need to function. The type, quantity, and quality of this fuel are all important. However, everything else matters as well, such as our sleep, breathing, physical activity, emotions, stress, and lifestyle.

By understanding more about these factors that affect the brain, we can unlock our potential for living a more joyful life, feeling physically well, and being mentally inspired.

Contents

1. Feeding Your Brain

Discover how foods can help your body stay in balance. It's important to remember that your body's needs change over time, so pay attention to its signals and take care of it properly as you go through this ongoing process called life.

This book is an introduction to the connection between food, the brain, and the chemistry that influences emotions. Think of it as a guide to help you improve your mental potential and happiness levels.

Inside, you will find theories and practical guidelines to help you integrate new habits and principles into your daily routine.

However, you don't need to do it all at once in practice. Making just small gradual changes maintained in the long-term is often the key to living a healthier life and preventing disease.

Remember that, in the end, consistency and persistence are the most important factors in creating a new lifestyle.

Food has an impact on your moods, emotions, and brain performance, altering the chemistry within you.

Consider this question: To what extent do physical conditions affect your moods and attitude?

There are numerous factors that influence the health of the brain and nervous system, impacting moods, cognitive abilities, sleep quality, and creativity.

The ability to solve problems, see the bigger picture, rearrange concepts to create new ones, and feel inspired could also be related to what happens inside the brain. The neurological system is interconnected with the rest of the body, enabling a two-way communication and triggering reactions and responses.

While our experience and perception of life are not only physical—we are more than a body—, it is important to see the influence of our physical health on it. Moreover, true holistic health also requires alignment and harmony between both our physical and spiritual selves.

This book focuses on the nutrition and lifestyle factors that physically support and impact the brain, without disregarding all the other aspects— existential or emotional—that also affect our experiences, and the importance of working with them.

Consider using these guidelines to complement your existing knowledge and determine what you currently need most. If you are interested in health, brain, and body science, this book might be suitable for you.

Remember, the point is to become healthier and happier. Take steps to improve without pressure or worry, as these won't make you feel better. You will not be healthier by adding additional stress, so just do your best at each moment, and be nice to yourself.

Don't settle for low energy as the norm. It might be common, but it's not natural. Uncover the root causes of your low energy, challenge old assumptions and habits, and improve your well-being and quality of life. Nobody else can do it for you.

2. Nourishment for Joy

Can emotional states affect the body?
Can physical states affect your emotional well-being?

2.1. Food for harmony

The food you eat and don't eat can impact your stress and energy levels. Although these are not the only factors, your ability to thrive in life is also linked to your overall health. For example, what happens in your gut affects hormonal levels, which in turn impact your nerves, moods, and therefore, happiness level.

Could an issue in the intestines be the reason for your low energy? Yes, it could be. However, it might also be something else. It is difficult to trace back the root causes of those symptoms and imbalances.

The best solution is often to start creating the conditions to resolve or prevent these imbalances. Don't become obsessed with the past; instead, learn from it and continue on your path.

Consider ha everything in nature moves toward a state of harmony, and beauty lies there. Every movement tends to find an equilibrium, which will change again and again, while life unfolds itself.

Forces interact to balance each other. Chaos eventually falls into order and rearranges itself for another scenario, another equilibrium, and another expression of beauty. Everything is always in motion.

All you nourish yourself with will create either chaos or order, affecting your physical and emotional states, as your body seeks to restore balance again. By paying closer attention to your body's signals, you will likely become more aware of its needs and better recognise those signs.

Understanding how to interpret your body's signals can help you comprehend the impact of food, habits, and other factors of your well-being. This knowledge has the potential to significantly improve your quality of life. Think of your body as being made by billions of living parts, with their harmony being essential for the proper functioning of the entire system.

Support your overall well-being and each part of your body with your choices, and trust in its ability to rebalance itself.

Not another set of rules

Don't think of this information as rules to follow or new doctrines that will control you or restrict you from your spontaneity and enjoyment. You probably already encounter enough of those in modern society.

Instead, this knowledge aims to help you understand your body better and encourage you to make small positive changes.

Prioritise emotional well-being and activities that bring you joy, as without that joy, we are not totally healthy. True health can only be achieved through a holistic approach.

Moreover, in challenging times, it might feel harder to try new things. However, this could be the time when you need it most. It can also be highly rewarding, and with motivation, you can surely move forward step by step.

Our preferences and taste change through new experiences, while our ideas and knowledge evolve. We can reeducate ourselves until we naturally crave healthy food and habits, as they will make us feel better.

Everything you do can put your body in a state of harmony or chaos. It's not really about following specific rules or diets, but nourishing yourself physically and mentally towards balance, adapting to each new context and your body's conditions.

2.2. Tendencies & habits

We can walk blindly, repeating the same patterns by not being aware of the reasons behind them and the invisible world of our feelings and thoughts. However, just because we can't see them it doesn't mean they don't exist or don't affect us. Their impact, both physically and mentally, may grow, demanding our attention and giving us signs of what we need. We must pay attention and be willing to listen.

Can emotions and thoughts affect the physical body? Absolutely. The relationship goes both ways. Physical and emotional well-being affect each other. Therefore, the last sections are dedicated to some activities to help get in touch and manage emotional states, such as mindfulness, breathing practices, movement, and art.

Eating habits, and all habits in general, are also closely related to emotions. It's common to change them when we are nervous or excited. Eating too quickly and stressed, consuming cheap junk food, or eating for comfort, may lead to imbalances and potential health problems in the long term.

Better choices can be made if we understand the consequences and motivations of our actions, the factors that shape our habits, and get in touch with ourselves. "The Psychology of Eating" section will help you consider the reasons for your choices and how to not perpetuate those that are no longer healthy.

We live in a constant state of evolution, always in motion, and absolutely capable of healthy transformations at all levels.

"We are what we eat"—yes, but not only. For example, we are also what we breathe and think. However, our food clearly impacts our energy levels, the brain, and all cognitive functions.

2.3. What if...

Feeling better and healthy is possible and worthwhile. However, this requires making different choices, one step at a time. Being proactive about our health and life requires courage, as it involves making decisions and embracing new possibilities.

This may not always be easy, but it's probably the way to lifestyle transformations. To change our health, we need to change the way we live, and that includes also changing our thoughts.

It often requires realising the fragile nature of our ideas and assumptions, revisiting and broadening them, and expanding the limits of our perception.

Our thoughts have a significant impact on us, including at a physical level. Scientific studies have already proven this, but we don't need to wait for more research to re-confirm it. We can already see it in our own experience and apply it in practice.

Evolving, in a way, means dying, letting go of a part of your identity and discovering new interpretations of the world, inside and outside of you.

You can shape the narrative of your personal story, reframe the interpretation of events, embrace different perspectives, and view challenges as opportunities for growth, even physical ones.

What would you do if you could?

What if?...

...You could take steps to improve your health and you didn't feel merely like a victim of circumstances?

...You could feel good most days, wake up refreshed and full of energy, enjoy a restful sleep every night, and feel focused and inspired more often?

...Or just simply feel a bit better?

Wouldn't it be worth trying?

3. Behind Your Moods

Different levels of certain chemicals can induce feelings of stress or calm, increase mental power, create a sense of love, or cause confusion. This is the science of emotions.

Have you ever heard about the relationships between serotonin, dopamine, endorphins, motivation, inspiration, and joy? Adrenaline and energy levels? Melatonin and sleeping patterns? Yes, you most likely have.

All these chemicals are some of the factors to unlocking your physical potential to thrive, and your lifestyle can significantly impact them. For example, inadequate sleep can leave your body alert and anxious, potentially leading to rude reactions toward others.

Likewise, if an external stressor triggers anxious feelings in you, how you respond to that can either help your body to calm down or worsen the state. Deep breathing would help regulate your body, while consuming alcohol or sugary foods would further stress it.

Energy
Balance
Stability
Creativity
Motivation
Inspiration

B12
Omega 3
Glutamate
Vitamin D
Magnesium

Serotonin
Dopamine
Endorphins
Adrenalin
Melatonin
Estrogen

Your emotions can also be signs of physical states, underlying imbalances, or hormonal chaos. In many of such cases, remedies would include changes in your diet and lifestyle. And, there are always steps you can take to achieve a bit more physical balance.

4. The Ten Commandments

The ten commandments for the brain and nervous system are a collection of habits, activities, and foods to include in your daily life to maximise your potential and emotional well-being. You don't need to do them all at once, but one at a time and keep it consistently in the long-term until it becomes a new habit.

1. Good fats

Include some healthy fats daily and Omega-3 sources at least three times per week. E.g., salmon, sardines, tuna, walnuts, flaxseeds, chia seeds, avocado, nuts & seeds, and extra virgin olive oil.

2. Gut health

Take care of your microbiota by consuming fibre-rich foods and fermented foods for probiotics. E.g., yogurt, kefir, kimchi, pickles, tempeh, miso, sauerkraut, kombucha, and plenty of veggies.

3. B Vitamins

Incorporate foods rich in the B vitamin group—E.g., mushrooms, green leafy veggies, broccoli, egg yolks, avocados, whole grains, quinoa, chickpeas, beans, fish, and organic liver. Vegetarian and vegan diets need to consider including B12 supplements.

4. Natural foods

Reduce processed products and replace them with natural and nutrient-dense foods that contain no added artificial ingredients and often more nutrients. If you choose processed foods, check the label and understand what you are consuming.

5. Sugars

Minimise or eliminate refined and added sugars. Substitute them with natural alternatives like fruit, and use stevia as a healthy sweetener. Consume sweets foods with fibre, protein or good fats.

6. Emotions

Make nourishing food choices when feeling sad, lacking motivation, stressed, or having sleeping troubles. E.g., bananas, nuts, 75% dark chocolate, warm soups, Omega-3 fish, and herbal teas.

7. "Junk"

Avoid junk food. Replace cravings for sweet or greasy foods with nourishing choices, such whole-grain and legumes, and opt for more natural over ultra-processed foods. E.g., a hot cocoa with honey or stevia, nuts, seeds, nut butter, fruits, avocados, veggies, hummus, or eggs.

8. Spices

Use spices and herbs to boost your mood and add flavour instead of processed sauces. E.g., ginger, cinnamon, turmeric, cardamom, cloves, coriander, basil, cumin, rosemary, parsley, mint, chilies, and garlic.

9. Stimulants

Reduce stimulants like caffeine, but especially alcohol. Limit your coffee intake to about 1 to 2 cups per day and avoid it in the evening. Try ginger tea, green tea, or herbal drinks.

10. Be happy

Every day, breathe deeply, get direct sunshine in the morning, do some physical activity, feel grateful for something, and do some creative or fun activities.

5. Your Brain Chemistry

Everything in your body is interconnected. This means that your physical health also impacts your emotional and mental well-being, and vice versa. Let's start with what happens inside the brain.

5.1. Neurotransmitters

Neurotransmitters are chemicals that allow the communication between brain's cells (neurons) and the rest of the body.

They act as messengers; without them, neurons wouldn't be able to talk, and the brain would essentially be switched off. For example, in Alzheimer's, it has been seen that there is damage to neurons and a decrease in certain types of neurotransmitters related to memory and learning. In the case of some drugs and pain inhibitors, they impact the transmission and reception of specific neurotransmitters.

When neuroscientists investigate the brain, they observe the functions and life cycles of these neurotransmitters and neurons, and which factors affect them.

Millions of conversations happen between cells, with a constant flow of chemicals consuming most of your daily energy. They drive your body's functions and moods, beyond your conscious control. Moreover, these communications never stop. The brain is constantly active and working, also while sleeping.

The neurological system and the brain are complex and only partially understood. Also, we can't underestimate other factors that impact them, such as genetics, epigenetics, psychology, diet, lifestyle, and most probably, our thoughts.

Complex issues can be handled if divided into smaller parts, one at a time. Then, let's see simple examples of what you can do in practice about these factors.

5.2. Examples and factors

The important part is that you can help your body regulate the levels of these chemicals that impact your emotions through your lifestyle and choices, including your diet. Here's an overview of some key neurotransmitters and some of the factors that influence them.

Norepinephrine
Attention

Norepinephrine plays a key role in controlling moods, attention, motivation, and the ability to cope with stressful situations. You can help balance its levels by consuming regularly almonds, avocados, pumpkin seeds, and cocoa, as well as by engaging in activities like meditation, deep sleep, and physical exercise.

Oxytocin
Social bonding

Oxytocin, also known as the "love drug," is involved in social bonding and sexual reproduction. You can increase its levels by socialising, listening to music, hugging, kissing, cuddling, and practicing loving kindness.

Endorphins
Pain reliever

Endorphin is an abbreviation for "endogenous morphine"— morphine naturally produced in the body. It interacts with the brain receptors that reduce pain perception, which are the same receptors that morphine communicates with. The most immediate way to increase endorphin levels is through physical exercise.

GABA

Low levels of GABA can lead to increased anxiety and difficulty sleeping. Foods rich in B6, magnesium, and glutamine amino acid such as eggs, dairy, fish, chicken, beets, beans, whole grains, legumes, nuts, seeds, broccoli, spinach, mushrooms, and cocoa can assist the body to produce GABA. Additionally, activities like yoga, meditation, walking in nature, journaling, and physical exercise can also help.

Acetylcholine

Acetylcholine is crucial for voluntary muscle coordination and memory. You can increase its levels by consuming avocados, almonds, yolks, full-fat dairy, and oily fish.

Serotonin

Serotonin has various positive effects, including producing calm and antidepressant effects, reducing headaches and migraines, aiding in addiction recovery, and impacting learning, energy, sleeping cycles, appetite, social behaviour, and menopause symptoms.

Dopamine

Dopamine is the main chemical responsible for feelings of motivation, satisfaction, reward, pleasure, and alertness. For example, it is released in the brain when you receive a reward or recognition, eat your favourite food, or scroll on social media.

The body needs specific components to produce these neurotransmitters. For instance, dopamine production relies on the amino acid tyrosine, and serotonin depends on the amino acid tryptophan. The tables below show some food groups particularly rich in those nutrients.

Dopamine: Tyrosine

Legumes: beans (kidney and black beans), split peas, chickpeas, and lentils

Grains: oats and rice

Seeds: pumpkin and sesame

Nuts: peanuts and almonds

Meat: turkey, pork, chicken, and beef

Fish/seafood: salmon, tuna, sardines, and shrimp

Eggs: egg whites

Dairy: yogurt, kefir, milk, and cheese

Soy: tofu and soybeans

Also, in bananas, avocados, spirulina, and cocoa

Serotonin: Tryptophan

Legumes: beans (small white beans), lentils, and chickpeas

Grains/cereals: oats, wheat, quinoa, and rice

Seeds: sunflower, sesame, chia, and pumpkin seeds

Eggs: egg whites

Fish/seafood: tuna, halibut, salmon, trout, sardines, crab scallops, and octopus

Meat: beef, turkey, and chicken

Soy: soybeans and tofu

Dairy: yogurt, milk, and cheese

Also, in cocoa, spirulina, and dried dates

6. List of Brain Essentials

Here are the lists of beneficial foods for brain health and well-being. Use them as references while you slowly put all this into practice. Theory is interesting, but it can lead to frustration without application.

However, making too many changes at once is often not sustainable. Therefore, choose only 2 to 3 foods, alternate between them regularly, and keep them in sight and accessible in your kitchen. Try new products every few weeks and aim for consistency in the long term.

Gut	Veggies & Fruits	B Vitamins	Omega 3
Kimchi	Leafy greens	Mushrooms	Flax seeds
Kefir	Spinach, kale	Quinoa	Walnuts
Yogurt	Broccoli	Eggs	Chia seeds
Kombucha	Collards	Beans	Hemp seeds
Tempeh	Brussel sprouts	Lentils	Salmon
Miso	Avocados	Chickpeas	Sardines
Sauerkraut	Berries	Seeds	Mackerel
Bone broth	Bananas	Nuts	Tuna
Aloe vera	Seaweed	Seafood & fish	Seafood
Honey		Organic liver	Cod liver oil

Other condiments and factors

Ginseng	Olive oil	Sleep & rest	Reduce:
Turmeric	Ashwagandha	Gratitude	Stress
Ginger	Green tea	Reading	Alcohol
Cinnamon	Sunlight	Creativity	Refined oils / Refined sugar
Cocoa	Movement	Art	Toxins

The next time you argue with someone who has excessive irritability or anxiety, instead of taking it personally, consider that such reaction could be the consequence of many different conditions and situations, including underlying physical imbalances.

Problems in the gastrointestinal tract or a poor diet, possibly originated from lack of sleep, chronic stress, deficiencies due to intolerances, lack of knowledge, or even economic limitations, could also be the reasons of those health issues and emotional distress.

However, it is not always related to imbalances or problems. It can also be due to the natural rhythm of each person, like it happens for women due to their cyclical nature, often neglected, or children with higher sensitivity, often misunderstood. Being aware of this can lead you not to take words personally, not to stand in judgment but to offer a better understanding, not to have a closed attitude but a receptive one, and therefore, to change the course of events.

This also applies to understanding yourself. The next time you experience emotional troubles, anxiety, or irritability, consider that your physical state may be playing a role in how you cope with them, even in your perception of them. This way you can also be more compassionate with yourself. Have a few good nights of sleep, eat well, and go for a walk before engaging in an argument, making a false conclusion, or taking important decisions.

7. The Brain is Mostly Fat

Fat has often received a negative reputation, but it is actually essential for the body. Although many want to lose it, we cannot live without it, especially the brain. The brain is primarily composed of fat, and it also plays a vital role in its development and maintenance.

60 %

of the brain is fat

If the brain does not get enough fat, it cannot function properly. However, the type, source, and quantity matter. The so-called "bad fats" are mainly refined and industrially created, such as refined oils and hydrogenated trans fats.

Reconsider the myth that fat is generally bad and learn why the body needs it so much. Question the associations made in the past about it, like the idea that low-fat processed products are healthier. Those past ideas primarily came from the food business and marketing campaigns without considering their impact on our health.

Healthy fats have essential roles in maintaining brain structure and performance, forming cell membranes and producing hormones, facilitating cell communication, regulating neurotransmitter functions, supporting the immune system, and more. Imbalances in the intake of these fats can have significant implications for overall health.

7.1. Types of fats

Foods with healthy fats, such as walnuts and sardines, have properties to help with attention and memory retention. However, it's important to maintain a consistent long-term approach for these foods and lifestyle choices to be effective as preventive measures.

Types and ratios

There are two main groups of natural fats: saturated and unsaturated, and neither group is inherently bad. Both are required in the right proportions, but modern diets often fail to maintain this balance.

For example, the proportion of saturated and Omega-6 fats in modern diets is often higher than what the human body needs.

This imbalance is attributed to the excessive quantity of these fats in many ultra-processed foods, as well as diets too high in fatty meats. These fats are often used to prolong the product's shelf life, solidify products, or enhance palatability. This also makes ultra-processed foods easy to overeat and can lead to food cravings and overconsumption.

Essential fatty acids

Essential fatty acids (EFAs) are the types of unsaturated fats that the body cannot produce and must obtained from food. There are two main EFAs: ALA or alpha-linolenic acid (Omega 3) and LA or linoleic acid (Omega 6), which have opposite effects.

Nowadays, the intake of Omega 6 is significantly higher, around 16 to 20 times more than what the body needs. To get an idea of what this represents, in the past when there were not ultra-processed foods, the ratio was close to 1:1, which is considered the ideal standard.

Therefore, in practice, modern diets are typically too high in Omega 6, and most people would benefit from increasing their intake of Omega-3 fats.

7.3. Tips for modern times

In modern times, some key considerations regarding fats include the balance of the Omega 6 and Omega 3 ratio, the quality of food, avoiding trans fats and ultra-processed foods, and checking food labels to understand what we are consuming.

The quality of food

The nutritional content of foods depends a lot on the origin—the way the food has been grown, the minerals in the soil, the water, the fertiliser, and the weather.

Take tomatoes, for example. If tomatoes are artificially grown with chemicals, they may end up looking like tomatoes, but they might lack the exact nutrients. For those nutrients to grow, they need certain conditions of water, soil, sun, and time.

Moreover, these chemicals can contaminate the plant, adding substances that are not beneficial for the body. As research has shown, many pesticides can have harmful effects on health.

Although there are differing opinions on the actual nutritional difference between organic and non-organic foods, there is general consensus about the adverse impact of certain pesticides on health.

In order to minimise this impact, be aware that that fruits and vegetables without hard peels are most contaminated by pesticides, such as strawberries, apples, pears, blueberries, kale, and spinach. Wash them properly, peel them, or buy them organic.

And the same applies to animal products and eggs—they are affected by how they are fed and grown. For instance, caged chicken eggs have lower nutrient density compared to eggs from free-range chickens, and chickens fed with a diet high in Omega 3 lay Omega 3-rich eggs. Even the colour and taste of the yolks, meat, and milk depend on how the animal was fed and treated.

Food labels list "total fats" and categorise them into saturated and polyunsaturated types. The overall fat content listed as "total value" does not mean much; it's important to know the type and quantity. This is given as grams per serving size or as the percentage of the recommended daily value (RDV or DV).

It's this last value (RDV) that is most meaningful. For example, if a product claims to contain Omega 3 but the quantity is less than 5 percent of the DV, it's a bit of a scam. However, if it provides 50 percent of your daily dosage, then it is a great source.

Be aware of false claims to make products look healthier, especially on the front package. Adopt the good habit to always turn the package and read the label.

Omega 3 and Omega 6 have opposing effects, and most foods contain both in different amounts. Omega 6 is an inflammatory agent and coagulant, and although this may not sound beneficial, it's needed in the right proportion. However, Omega 6 deficiency is very rare. Symptoms can be skin and hair problems, dry eyes, poor wound healing, and persistent infections.

The problem usually lies in an excess of Omega 6. To reduce it, consider consuming fewer products with sunflower, corn, soybean, or cottonseed oil. Use ghee, butter, olive oil, or unrefined coconut oil in your kitchen. In addition to this, consume more Omega-3 fish an other food sources, like walnuts, flaxseed, or their cold-pressed oils in order to balance out your Omegas ratio intake.

Omega 3 claims

When a package says it contains Omega 3, it may not be significant if the quantity is too small. Always check the nutritional content to find out, and this advice applies to other nutritional claims as well.

Advertising claims depend on each country's regulations, so it's important to double-check the labels. If a food does contain Omega 3, the label will indicate how much DHA, EPA, or "other" (often ALA) it contains. Note that ALA is Omega 3 from plant origin and is less easily absorbed. Moreover, try to obtain nutrients from food, as this is the best form for the body to absorb and utilise them. However, if also complementing it with supplements, be aware that Omega 3 is prone to go rancid. Check for any unusual smell, old dates, and if it contains antioxidants like vitamin E to help preserve it. Also, confirm the quantity of DHA and EPA (not ALA), and check for unnecessary additives.

Trans fats

Trans fats are mainly industrially produced to prolong the shelf life of foods and convert liquid fats into a solid form. They were commonly used in industrial pastries, baked goods, and ultra-processed foods. However, research has shown that they are detrimental to health, leading some countries to ban their use, such as Denmark. The advice is to avoid trans fats, also known as hydrogenated fats on food labels.

Hydrogenated fats

Hydrogenated or trans fats may be found in margarine spreads, shortenings, and some types of cakes, cookies, and pastries.

Any "hydrogenated" or "partially hydrogenated" oil in the ingredients list indicates the presence of trans fat, even if not specified on the nutritional value. Also, note that food labels list their ingredients in order of their quantity. Therefore, if trans fat appears early on the list, it indicates a high amount of trans fat in that food.

7.4. Omega 3 dossier

Brain and mental well-being

Omega 3 is essential for the brain's structure and mental performance and for creating new neurotransmitters, which are the messengers in the brain. Research has shown that neurons can be regenerated, contrary to previous assumptions, and good fats are related to this process called neurogenesis.

Low intakes of Omega 3 can lead to a predisposition to depression, anxiety, behavioural conditions, poor concentration, and certain diseases such as early dementia, Alzheimer's, or Parkinson's.

Anti-inflammatory properties

Studies has indicated that Omega 3 has properties as part of the prevention and treatment of inflammation, auto-immune conditions, arthritis, and joint problems.

However, it's important to note that real benefits are gained through a balanced lifestyle rather than relying solely on one remedy. Everything is interconnected. For instance, taking Omega-3 supplements in a diet high in processed and junk foods does not compensate. Additionally, you are likely to start feeling the effects only after consistently practicing these habits for a certain period. This means that rarely eating walnuts or salmon will not make any difference or effectively help in the prevention of disease. Consistency with habits is an essential factor in establishing and improving your health.

Types of Omega 3

Omega 3 comes in different types: EPA and DHA, which are mainly found in oily fish, and ALA, which comes from vegetarian sources like walnuts. The body needs to convert ALA into DHA or EPA in order to use it, but the conversion rate is low.

Origin matters

Most research on Omega 3 health benefits refers to EPA and DHA from animal origins. Only a fraction of the ALA present in plants and nuts is converted into EPA and DHA by the body. Studies also suggest that Omega 3 from fish may be more effective than supplements for many health claims. If you are not vegetarian, the recommendation is to include oily fish in your diet about three times a week. For vegetarians or vegans, it's important to consume generous amounts of plant-based sources and consider the following recommendations.

What if you are vegetarian?

The efficiency of converting ALA to EPA and DHA depends on age and overall health. A balanced diet and lifestyle are necessary along with consuming enough Omega 3 for your specific needs. Deficiencies in certain minerals and vitamins, as well as an excess of Omega 6, saturated fats, and trans fats, can decrease this conversion. Reduce these fats and increase your Omega 3 intake by including ground flaxseeds, walnuts, chia seeds, or their corresponding unrefined oils in your diet. You can also consider a microalgae Omega 3 supplement as a recommended EPA and DHA plant source.

7.5. What does it mean in practice?

The fat in food is always a combination of different fatty acids, with one type being more predominant, which determines the properties and classification. Therefore, the foods listed below contain a variety of fats and are particularly rich in the following types.

To assess your diet, consider whether you are consuming fats from each of the following three groups in equal proportions. You may need to include more Omega 3 and monounsaturated fats while reducing your consumption of saturated fats and Omega 6.

However, keep in mind that the ideal proportions may vary based on your unique circumstances. It's important not to follow general recommendations without analysing your health, diet, age, lifestyle, personal conditions, and any other specific requirements.

Saturated	Monounsaturated
Coconut oil	Extra virgin olive oil
Coconut milk	Cold pressed sesame oil
Butter and ghee	Nuts
Hard cheese	Seeds
Cream	Avocados
Fatty meat	Egg yolks
Cured meat	Oily fish
Cocoa	Seafood
Most bakery and fast foods	Olives

Polyunsaturated

Omega 3

Oily fish and seafood

Salmon

Mackerel

Sardines

Tuna

Anchovies

Herring

Trout

Nuts and seeds

Flaxseeds

Walnuts

Chia seeds

Hemp seeds

Cold-pressed nuts oils

Supplements

Microalgae & fish oil

Natto (a soy-based Japanese fermented dish)

Omega 6

Refined vegetable oils

Sunflower

Corn

Soybean

Cottonseed

Peanut

Sunflower

Sunflower seeds or butter

Cured processed meats like salami or pepperoni

Most industrial cakes, cookies, and snacks made with vegetable oils

Ultra-processed products

Potato and corn chips

Fast and junk foods

8. The Energy Vitamins

B vitamins are considered to be directly related to happiness, motivation, the capacity to handle stress, concentration, focus, and memory retention.

Deficiencies in these vitamins over a long period can result from poor diets or physical issues that lead to poor absorption. These deficiencies can lead to physical imbalances that affect mood, mental performance, and overall neurological well-being. And the truth is that when basic physical needs are not met, coping with life's stressors can become more difficult.

Traditionally, such conditions have often been overlooked or misunderstood, but now you have a better understanding of them. Remember that overall lifestyle and diet can impact your capacities and quality of life.

Nuts and seeds
Mushrooms
Beans, lentils, chickpeas, oats
Greens, broccoli, spinach
Fish, salmon, mussels, clams
Fruits, bananas, avocados
Eggs, dairy
Organic meats, organ meats

B_1 or thiamine
B_2 or riboflavin
B_3 or niacin
B_5 or pantothenic acid
B_6 or pyridoxine
B_7 or biotin
B_9 folic acid
B_{12} or cobalamin

B vitamins act as keys that unlock energy, the sensation to be motivated, and brain potential. They are essential for energy production and brain function.

8.1. The main energy vitamins

All B vitamins are important for brain functions and energy production. Concretely, B6, B9 (folic acid), and B12 are particularly important for cognitive well-being and maintaining the right balance of the brain and nervous system chemicals.

B6 or pyridoxine

B6 is required for energy production, brain function, and a healthy immune system. It also plays a role in hormone and neurotransmitter formation.

For instance, B6 is linked to serotonin, a chemical responsible for feelings of happiness. It is also involved in red blood cell production, impacts energy levels, and provides a sense of vitality.

B9 or folate

B9 or folate primarily helps in making new cells and providing building blocks for the body, including DNA replication during cells regeneration. It is also critical during pregnancy for the fetal brain development.

Deficiencies

All B vitamins have similar imbalance symptoms, mostly related to the nervous system and mental performance.

Some examples are mood swings, decreased mental sharpness, memory and concentration issues, irritability, weakness, fatigue, and confusion. However, these symptoms can also have other causes, such as lack of sleep or excessive psychological stress. It's important to note if they appear while all the other life conditions remain the same to understand the real causes.

B vitamins are also vital for the nervous system and brain development during pregnancy and early childhood, which can significantly impact adult health later in life.

8.2. The famous B12

The B12 vitamin is a common concern for those following plant-based diets because it is primarily found in animal sources. The B12 stores in the body can take some years to get depleted, even when it is not consumed through the diet.

B12, also known as cobalamin, is crucial for the nervous system, hormones and neurotransmitter production, red blood cell formation, and DNA synthesis.

It also plays a role in the metabolism of fats and proteins or in producing energy from these nutrients. Therefore, fatigue and weakness are among the initial most common symptoms of B12 deficiency.

Moreover, like other B vitamins an as previously explained, B12 is vital for brain and nervous system development during pregnancy and the first years of life.

The body can't produce B12, but it can store it, especially in the liver. These stores can last for some years before being depleted, even if B12 is no longer present in the diet. However, it is not recommended to only rely on B12 stores.

During digestion, B12 gets combined with a substance called "intrinsic factor" in the stomach and is absorbed in the small intestine. Therefore, individuals with stomach issues and the elderly, whose bodies may not produce enough of this essential intrinsic factor, may need to monitor their B12 levels.

Common symptoms of B12 deficiency include fatigue, sleeping problems, nervousness, poor concentration, and a tingling sensation in the hands or feet. It is advisable for vegetarians, the elderly, and individuals with stomach issues to monitor their B12 levels.

Deficiency

Deficiency symptoms are usually related to mental performance and energy levels. These symptoms can include brain fog, weakness, unexplainable fatigue, nervousness, sleeping problems, irritability, and poor concentration.

A common and early symptom, particularly in older individuals, is a tingling or numbness in the hands, feet, or legs.

People at risk

People at risk for B12 deficiency include the elderly, individuals with ulcers or stomach surgery, and vegetarians or vegans since B12 is mainly found in animal products.

B12 injections should be taken every few months when the body cannot absorb it from dietary sources. For individuals following a vegan diet, they are advised to include foods fortified with B12 and a B12 supplement.

8.3. What does it mean in practice?

Instead of searching for foods high in every B vitamin, which would be very complicated, focus on food groups with high B vitamin content. Specific lists for B6, B9, and B12 can also be found in following pages for your reference.

You can place them in a visible place at the beginning to remind you to include them in your daily choices. Try to make the practice as simple as possible to create new long-term habits.

Sources

B Vitamins

Green leaves

Spinach

Broccoli

Egg yolks

Mushrooms

Whole grains

Lentils, beans,
and chickpeas

Nuts and seeds

Avocados

Oily fish

Oysters, clams,
and mussels

Fortified
nutritional yeast

Quality meat

Organic liver

Food groups

Fortunately, in practice, you don't need to know which specific foods contain each vitamin, which would be very impractical. All B vitamins are typically found in the same types of foods, making it easier for you.

This list gives the main food groups rich in all B vitamins, which is important to remember in your daily life.

Food quality

As previously explained, the origin matters. The quality of food depends on how they have been grown—the soil, water, time, and chemicals. As a consequence, this will also impact the nutrient content.

Additionally, the origin of the food matters for other reasons, such as potential environmental contamination during the transport, and supporting local economies when you consume directly from them.

As a general guideline, the more you can consume locally, seasonally, and naturally, the better. This means better for both your body and the environment.

Sources

The following lists of vitamin sources indicate how much percentage one cup of food gives of the recommended daily value (DV). For example, one cup of bananas can approximately give 20% of vitamin B6 recommended daily.

B12 (Cobalamin)	B9 (Folate)	B6 (Pyridoxine)
Liver >100%	Chickpeas>100%	Sunflower seeds 94%
Oysters >100%	Liver 90%	Pistachos 69 %
Mussels >100%	Lentils 90%	Chickpeas 55%
Crab >100%	Pinto beans 74%	Dried fruit 50 %
Sardines >100%	Asparagus 65%	Tuna 50%
Mackerel >100%	Spinach 65%	Turkey 50%
Fortified cereals 100%	Beets 34%	Beef 45%
Trout 90%	Papayas 29%	Chicken 40%
Salmon 80%	Avocados 28%	Salmon 35%
Tuna 42%	Broccoli 26%	Halibut 35%
Haddock 30%	Okra 25%	Avocados 33%
Milk 18%	Green peas 25%	Potatoes 20%
Yogurt 23%	Peanuts 22%	Walnuts 25%
Beef 23%	Sunflower seeds 22%	Spinach 22%
Cheese 16%	Cauliflower 14%	Bananas 20%
Chicken 5%	Green beans 10%	Tofu 5%
	An egg yolk 6%	

9. Your Gut: The Second Brain

This sentence adds another dimension to the famous saying, "You are what you eat," by emphasising that it's not just our diet that matters, but also what the body can absorb and do with that food.

Trillions of bacteria in the gut have roles in digestion and "communicate" with the brain through a complex two-way signalling pathway. The balance of all the bacteria in your body, called the microbiota, affects your overall well-being, including hormonal levels, energy, immune system, and cognitive conditions. Although this field is relatively new, the importance of gut health cannot be overstated.

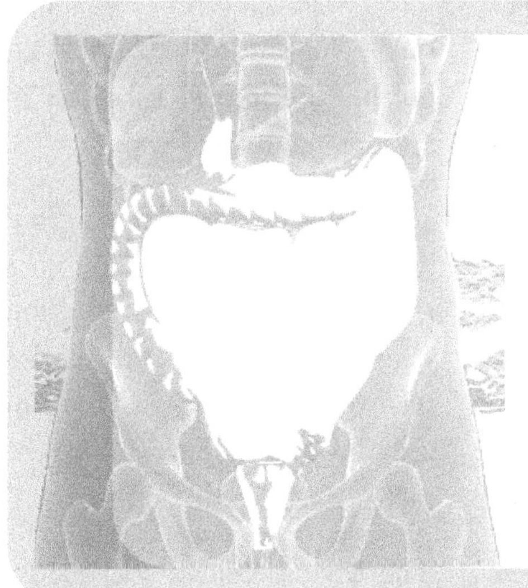

Both physical and cognitive symptoms could be related to imbalances in the colonies of bacteria in your body, also called microbiota. Additionally, in some cases, dietary and lifestyle changes are the most important factors for recovery or healing.

Gut health and microbiota impact overall health, including the brain and nervous system. It's not a surprise that the origin of "gut feelings" expression is rooted in the interaction between the brain, the gut, emotions, and the microbiota.

9.1. Inside your second brain

Everything is interconnected; even what you consider just your body is hosting many other lives inside and needs them to function. Around 500 to 1000 different species of bacteria live in the intestines, which play crucial roles for our well-being and cognitive health. We need those bacteria to live in a symbiotic relationship.

Human microbiota: The non-human cells in you

The human body has trillions of microorganisms from thousands of varieties that are non-human cells, which means that they have different DNA from ours. The mouth and the gut are the parts with the most abundance of these microorganisms.

This group of microorganisms is referred to as the human microbiota, and its composition varies from person to person. Those differences can influence the predisposition of each person to develop certain diseases.

While these microorganisms have very important roles, issues can often arise when their balance is out of their healthy ranges. Such imbalances can lead to complications such as obesity, liver disease, allergies, diabetes, behavioural issues, and autoimmune conditions. And although the exact causes of those diseases are most often unknown, research suggests that gut health can play a key role in uncovering the answers.

Which factors determine this? The composition of the gut flora is established during the first years of life and tends to remain relatively stable. However, it can also be altered later in life by dietary and lifestyle factors.

The colonisation of the gut by microorganisms begins at birth. Factors such as the method of delivery (cesarean section or natural birth), and whether a baby is breastfed can impact the types and balances of different gut bacteria during adulthood.

The early years are crucial for preventing possible problems later on, as it's like building the foundations of health. Bear this in mind if you are in charge of little people. And if you are not, it doesn't matter what your age is now; you can always improve!

The second brain

Have you ever heard the traditional expression "to feel nauseous" or "to feel butterflies in the stomach"? There is a nervous system in your belly and it contains over 100 million nerve cells and 400 million neurons.

It's called the enteric nervous system and is embedded in the lining covering the digestive system, playing a key role in controlling digestive processes. For example, approximately 90 percent of the body's total serotonin and 50 percent of dopamine are located in the gut. This amazing fact could change the way you take care of your belly and the digestive system.

In addition to this, our attitude in life, thoughts, social environment, and the brain's ability to adapt, determine our emotional well-being too. However, physical health and different chemical balances are also factors in this equation of our ability to handle challenges or retain information. For instance, we can cope with a stress better if being well-rested rather than sleep deprived.

The capacity of the brain to change as a result of experience is called neuroplasticity. It is related to the ability of neurons and neurotransmitters to take

The early years of life are a critical period, as it is when the intestinal flora rapidly develops and will usually stay moderately stable during adulthood. However, you can also improve it throughout your life, regardless of what happened before.

different paths, form new connections, and create networks. This is crucial to view situations from different perspectives, see the whole picture, have empathy, or feel connected to life. In other words, it impacts our capacity to experience life and happiness.

Experience is a significant factor influencing our neuroplasticity. It shapes our neural circuits, making them more functional and even creating new ones. Traveling, reading, engaging in art, studying, socialising, having positive conversations, music, changing our routines, stepping out of our comfort zone, and movement all help to keep our brains "young."

This is another reason why genuine health is holistic—everything is interconnected. If you are contemplating changing your diet but it's challenging, start with activities that you enjoy, like dancing or walking, which will also boost your motivation. Start with what you can and build it up from there.

Gut-brain axis

The gut-brain axis (GBA) refers to the communication between the central nervous system and the digestive tract, including the two-way communication pathways between the brain and the nervous system localised in the gut. Moreover, the microbial communities in the gut also influence these interactions.

Recent studies focus on how changes in the GBA may offer potential therapies for conditions such as autism, Asperger's, Parkinson's, and anxiety, which are not yet fully understood.

There is also emerging research suggesting that treatments targeting gut microbiota could play a role in psychiatry. During the "Microbiota for Health World Summit" in Paris in 2017, with more than 400 scientists, they replaced the famous "you are what you eat" with "you are what your gut microbes do with what you eat." Some examples presented were about gut-brain communication, specific probiotics to help alleviate depression, new therapies based on diet, and the impact of gut microbe on immune conditions, obesity, intolerances, chronic inflammation, skin problems, hormonal imbalances, obesity, anxiety, and IBS.

Unhealthy gut

An unhealthy gut can lead to various health issues, as previously explained. Treatment should be holistic, addressing stress levels, emotional well-being, alcohol consumption, smoking, sleep quality, exposure to toxins, and diet.

One example of an unhealthy gut condition is leaky gut syndrome, where the intestinal lining is damaged, causing increased permeability. This allows harmful bacteria and toxins to enter the bloodstream, and potentially impacting overall health.

However, there is much debate surrounding this topic. The key takeaway is that regardless of contradicting opinions or interpretations of research studies, results show the importance of gut health for overall well-being.

If you suspect that you may have an unhealthy gut, it's essential to be patient before rushing into a diagnosis since symptoms like fatigue can be related to other factors. Take your time to identify the underlying causes. You can then follow the recommendations in this book for a few months while discarding other possible issues, and consult a specialist for a personalised guidance.

The body has an incredible capacity to heal itself. If you are experiencing symptoms of imbalances, approach your healing holistically and be patient, consistent, and curious. Quick solutions are often not real or lasting solutions.

9.2. Gut imbalances

The brain and the gastrointestinal system are directly connected. Imbalances in one can impact the other. Intestinal problems can cause anxiety, stress, or emotional imbalance, just as anger and resentment can trigger symptoms in the gut. You may have heard that stress can cause many diseases, and disease can also cause a lot of stress.

The following are examples of potential symptoms and conditions that could benefit from making dietary changes to improve the gut microbiota balance and the gut lining. Note that these conditions require further understanding and can vary significantly from person to person, even if diagnosed with the same name.

While gut microbiota treatment shows promising potential, making improvements to your lifestyle and diet is also beneficial. Every positive change counts, so start with what you can and build up from there.

Symptoms	Pathologies
Difficulties coping with stress	New allergies or intolerances
Headache and brain fog	Autism and Asperger's
Food sensitivities	Childhood behaviour issues
Chronic fatigue	Acne, psoriasis, and eczema
Attention deficit	Rheumatoid arthritis Autoimmune
Mood swings	disorders
Hyper activity	Crohn's disease, IBS Fibromyalgia
Gas and bloating	and spondylitis Asthma
Joint pain	Alzheimer's and Parkinson's
Skin issues	Diabetes type 2

9.3. The roles of good bacteria

What do "good" bacteria do for you?

"Communicating" with the brain

The gut-brain axis is the signalling pathway between the gut and the central nervous system. The gut flora plays important roles in these complex interconnections—400 times more messages come from the microbiome to the brain than from the brain to the body. For instance, it can activate pathways between the gut and the brain, improving brain function and nervous system conditions. As a result, research is exploring the potential use of certain bacteria as part of the treatment for specific nervous system conditions.

Defending against harmful organisms

Bacteria play a crucial role in protecting the surface of the intestines, serving as a barrier against toxins and harmful bacteria. Additionally, 70-80% of immune cells reside in the gut, highlighting the intricate relationship between the intestinal microbiota and the immune system.

Turning dietary fibre into crucial fats

Furthermore, bacteria ferment and convert fibre into important fatty acids that play significant roles in overall health. For example, these fatty acids help in the production of immune cells, supporting the body's defence against diseases.

Assisting the digestion of big molecules

Bacteria play a crucial role in helping the body digest large food molecules. For instance, some bacteria break down carbohydrates into forms that the body can utilise. Another example is the dietary fibre, also explained in this section, which is transformed into essential types of fats.

Producing certain vitamins

Bacteria also aid in the production of essential vitamins such as B and K. This means that the body can synthesise or make certain vitamins from the foods we eat and with the help of these bacteria.

Helping nutrient absorption

Furthermore, bacteria assist in the absorption of important nutrients like magnesium, calcium, and iron. If these nutrients are not effectively absorbed, they won't reach the bloodstream and the body will not be able to use them. Therefore, the quality of our diet is not only determined by what we eat but also by what the body is able to absorb.

Recovering and rebalancing gut health is often one of the first steps in any process of healing or improving our diet. This also applies to supplements. It's important to focus on improving gut health before taking supplements in order to absorb them properly and maximise their benefits, avoiding wasting money.

9.4. What does it mean in practice?

Less of what damages the gut

Gut health can be damaged by antibiotics, NSAIDS, medications, pesticides, and inflammatory foods such as refined sugars, hydrogenated oils, artificial sweeteners, processed foods high in those ingredients, environmental toxins, stress, and emotions like resentment. For instance, many doctors nowadays warn against excessive use of medications due to their impact on liver and gut health. They also recommend probiotics or fermented foods after antibiotic use to help restore gut flora.

More of what heals the gut

Consider incorporating vegetables into your diet, including a variety of types and colours. They offer plenty of healthy properties and are high in fibre, which is one of the most beneficial nutrients for the gut. Other foods rich in dietary fibre are fruits, beans, legumes, nuts, and seeds, especially flax and chia. Additionally, bone broth, aloe vera, honey, pollen, propolis, papaya, digestive enzymes, and fermented foods are also recommended for their gut-healing properties.

Peace of mind

Peace of mind and mental well-being play crucial roles in gut health. Stress and repressed emotions can negatively impact our overall health, including the balance of gut microbiota.

Include probiotics and prebiotics

Probiotics are beneficial live bacteria that help in rebalancing the gut flora. You can obtain them from supplements or fermented foods—see the lists below.

However, if you consume probiotics alone between meals, some may not survive the stomach conditions and reach the gut, potentially perishing before getting to their final destination.

You can assist probiotics in their journey through the digestive system by combining them with foods rich in prebiotic fibre, such as fruits and vegetables.

Probiotics	Prebiotic
Kimchi	Apple cider vinegar
Sauerkraut	Onions and garlic
Kombucha	Oats, wheat, and bran
Kefir	Chicory root
Yogurt	Artichoke
Curd	Asparagus
Miso	Fruits
Tempeh	Leeks
Natto	Beans
Pickles	Barley
Sourdough	Cocoa
Raw-milk cheese	Flaxseeds
Raw-milk buttermilk	

10. Sugar & the Brain

Nowadays, it is widely recognised that consuming refined white sugar can have harmful effects, a fact you may have already heard many times. This chapter aims to explain this topic and emphasises the importance of finding a healthy balance in our choices.

First of all, it's important not to panic with so much conflicting information available. This can be overwhelming. The intention of this book is not to add more worries or make you overly picky about your food choices. Instead, it aims to increase your awareness of how your choices impact your life and your responsibility for your health. In real life, try to follow the guidelines with flexibility, and remember that balance is key. For instance, when it comes to refined sugar, you don't need to avoid all foods containing sugars, but it's important to be aware of thes negative effects and avoid excessive consumption. Sometimes, what is considered "normal" in society may be too much and harmful for our bodies.

Refined sugars

Excessive refined sugars can lead to addictions and have various negative effects including anxiety, cravings, learning difficulties, and early diabetes.

Natural sugars

On the other hand, natural sugars, which are found mostly in fruits and vegetables, can provide a healthier energy for the brain.

Glucose is the name for blood sugar and the brain needs it for energy. The brain is the most energy-demanding organ and it can use about a half of all the sugar energy in the body.

10.1. Blood sugar levels

Fluctuations in blood sugar levels can significantly impact how we feel throughout the day and our long-term health. This is an important consideration for anyone looking to improve their health. Following these guidelines can help regulate blood sugar, reduce sugar cravings, maintain stable energy levels throughout the day, achieve mental clarity, improve sleep, and promote overall health.

10.2. Sugar & the brain

The brain uses 20 percent of our daily energy intake, mainly from glucose, which is blood sugar. This means that sugar is necessary, but not all sugars have the same effect. Natural sugars found in vegetables and fruits provide the body with energy along with fibre and other essential nutrients. On the other hand, added sugars, such as those in sweetened drinks and baked goods, can lead to health issues if consumed in excess.

It's also about moderation with portion sizes. However, it's very easy to overeat these products. Sugar stimulates the release of neurotransmitters in the brain that are responsible for pleasure, and therefore, moderation can be difficult to apply and addictions could even happen. Moreover, excessive sugar consumption can also harm brain cells in a process called oxidative stress.

Sugar addiction is a real concern due to the excessive amount of added sugar in modern diets. The body becomes used to higher levels of this pleasure-inducing chemical in the brain, resulting in increased cravings and the need for more sugar. This can lead to symptoms such as mood swings, cravings, headaches, and irritability, which are often misinterpreted or even considered normal. This cycle can create a dependency on sugary foods, leading to further negative effects physically and emotionally.

10.3. Spikes & fatigue

Regulating blood sugar levels is essential in order to maintain consistent energy throughout the day without fatigue, brain fog, and mood swings.

Here's how it works: After food is absorbed, nutrients are released into the blood, causing glucose levels to rise. This can give a "sugar rush", making us feel excited. If we need energy at that moment, such as when we are working out or cycling, the sugar will be used and can improve performance. However, if we don't need the energy right away, the excess sugar will be stored or converted into fat, leaving us feeling tired and sleepy. This is the "sugar crash."

First, the extra sugar is stored in the liver and muscles as "glycogen reserves" to be used by the brain and the rest of the body when required. However, these reserves are small. Once they are full, the extra blood sugar is converted and stored as fat tissue. As a result, diets too high in sugar can likely lead to obesity, which is common nowadays. Modern diets often have more sugar than necessary for a sedentary lifestyle.

After the initial "sugar rush," there is a rapid drop in blood sugar levels, leading to tiredness, sleepiness, or brain fog. These feelings are often symptoms of unhealthy fluctuations in blood sugar levels. Consequently, maintaining more balanced blood sugar levels can lead to more consistent energy levels. In practice, this can be achieved through our dietary choices, food combinations, physical activity, and stress reduction.

Feeling tired during the day is not normal, even if it is sometimes common and accepted. If you already sleep well, consider applying the principles to regulate blood sugar levels —it may be an important underlying cause of your fatigue.

Here are some practical guidelines: sugar and simple carbohydrates make those levels rise rapidly, but when combined with fat, fibre, or protein, they rise more slowly and evenly. Too big meals can also make blood sugar levels spike higher and faster. Also, engaging in physical activity after eating can help prevent unhealthy spikes.

10.4. Diabetes & other risks

Diabetes is a condition in which blood sugar levels remain too high for extended periods, and the body is unable to regulate them properly. Normally, the body has a mechanism to adjust these levels using insulin or glucagon as needed. However, in diabetes, this mechanism doesn't work properly.

There are two primary types of diabetes: type 1 and type 2. Type 1 is an autoimmune disorder that involves a genetic predisposition and issues with the pancreas. Type 2 is often linked to lifestyle, diet, and environmental factors.

This means that type 2 diabetes can often be prevented with our choices through the years.

It's important to determine if you are in a pre-diabetes state to manage it or even reverse it. Uncontrolled long-term diabetes can eventually impact overall health, including the brain.

If you have had a diet too high in sugar or unhealthy irregular eating habits, you could get your fasting blood sugar levels checked. This is especially important for older adults, as these functions can naturally deteriorate with age.

Other risks

Here is a list of potential effects of consuming excessive amounts of sugar through the years: Increased risk of type 2 diabetes, cardiovascular problems, cognitive and learning deficits, growth of "bad" gut bacteria, and liver damage. In the case of liver damage, the symptoms could even deteriorate similarly to a liver damaged by alcohol.

Below are some practical suggestions for maintaining healthy blood sugar levels throughout your day and replacing refined sugar with healthier choices in your meals and snacks.

Sweet snacks replacements

Options for replacing sugary snacks with nutritious choices, which will also keep you feeling energised:

Fruits, nuts, seeds, nut butters, avocados, whole-grain crackers, veggie sticks with hummus or guacamole, rice crackers with pickles, sourdough with cream cheese (vegan or not), dark chocolate >75%, dates with walnuts, or hot cocoa with stevia.

Alternatives in recipes

Consider using naturally sweet foods in recipes to replace white sugar in your cooking and baking:

Dates, raisins, or other dried fruits give sweetness to any dish, including salads. Stevia, honey, raw palm, or coconut sugar are great natural sweeteners for any recipe or drink. And, starchy vegetables or fruits like beetroot, pumpkin, or bananas, are sweet and can provide a great consistency for baking and desserts.

Choosing low-GI foods

When choosing foods, consider the glycemic index (GI), which measures how fast the sugar in a specific food is released into the blood on a scale from 0 to 100.

Foods with lower GI provide more stable energy, while those with higher GI can lead to energy spikes and drops, accompanied by sleepiness, tiredness, and brain fog. If we have more stable energy, we can live actively instead of always being tired, reactively, or like in survival mode.

As a general guideline, vegetables have a low GI, fruits have a medium GI, most grains and bread have a higher GI, and most sweets and refined flours have the highest GI. However, the total GI of a meal depends on the food combination, and therefore, remember to always add fibre, protein, or good fat in your meals.

Sugar on food labels

Sugar used to be in most of processed foods, but nowadays, plenty of brands have reduced it and "sugar-free" products are becoming more popular. However, it's important to be cautious of false claims and always check product labels.

What are some sugar names on food labels?
Corn syrup, high-fructose corn syrup, fruit juice concentrate, maltose, dextrose, sucrose, honey, and maple syrup.

How much sugar is too much?
More than 22.5 grams of sugar per 100 grams is considered high, and less than 5 grams is considered low.

II. The Psychology of Eating

We have more reasons to eat than only for nourishment, although this should be the priority. Next time you grab a snack, ask yourself why you want to eat it. Understanding this can help you make better choices and recognise when you are truly hungry or what you really need at each moment. The way we treat our bodies and take care of ourselves also reflects how we approach life and all our other relationships. As traditional wisdom says, start working on yourself, and everything else will follow.

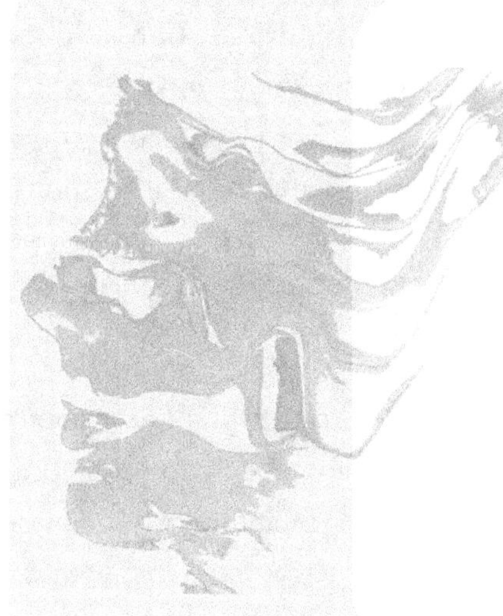

If a habit or assumption negatively impacts our well-being, it's important to question it and reeducate ourselves. We need to learn what the body needs, but simply knowing is most often not enough. Awareness of the factors that shape our habits and how we handle emotions is key to making lasting changes.

How did those habits start? What factors influence our routine, lifestyle, and food choices? Are they related to family, economic status, emotional states, social influence, or culture? How do we change the way we eat depending on how we feel? Why do we make certain unhealthy choices?

II.I. The reasons behind

Have you been rewarded or punished with food as a child? Have you used it to get the love or attention of someone? Do you remember the smell of cookies in your mum's kitchen? It's never just about food, as it's never only about the apparent reasons at first glance. There are always underlying and deeper motives that drive our decisions.

Sharing food brings undeniable pleasure and serves more functions than just nourishing the body, and that's okay. If we were purely functional, it would be boring, but without health, it is certainly more challenging. However, health can be simpler and we can make choices that prioritise our well-being while embracing its other functions.

Think of the cultural significance of food. It is related to concepts of wealth, social status, and beauty. For instance, in certain cultures, prolonged fasting is seen as a display of self-control, or feeding someone is a language of showing care. Food serves many more roles beyond only providing nourishment, and the industry around it has also made good profit from it. However, we can learn from all this.

First, it's important to question the reasons behind choices and habits, while learning about health and nutrition. These steps may seem obvious, but we often assume we know enough, which hinders further learning and makes us stuck in our limitations.

Then, observe yourself. Why do you repeat a habit that no longer serves you? Which situations and feelings trigger it? Do you act with awareness or do you repeat a pattern on autopilot? It can be difficult to accept the level of assumptions our lives may be based on, the consequences of that, and the possibility that this can change. Embracing change usually means letting go of something else. Otherwise, we are often reacting as slaves to our ideas, assumptions, or fears.

II.2. Knowledge is surely not enough

This is an invitation to question your beliefs, ideas, and assumptions while staying open to changing them when needed. Life makes us to be in constant evolution, but if we resist growing, we end up limited by the narrow scope of our own ideas. Expose yourself to knowledge, but also take time to quiet the inner noise and connect with yourself.

Understanding the reasons behind our choices will make it easier to transform habits and see more clearly what we really need. And, being aware of all the assumptions we constantly build our life on, will make them more flexible to evolve when needed.

Just the intention to reflect on this leads us to see underneath where the real drivers of our actions and emotions are. Consider that until we don't get in touch with the deeper layers of ourselves, we are somehow just reacting to them and not truly free. Then, stay honest and authentic with yourself. And consider that the choices we make today will impact both our quality of life and the lives of future generations, as we are always setting an example for others with our actions.

We can blindly repeat our beliefs, ideas, and habits, or take a step back to observe how they started and their current impact on us. Then, we can allow them to slowly change, based on whether they still serve us or not. It's also important to recognise the filters through which we perceive reality and their limitations. This way, we can transform our lifestyles and reinvent ourselves.

Flexibility and adaptability are also essential in this learning process. Change often involves letting go of something. It is a bit like dying, there is always a part of the old that fades away for the new to emerge. However, the new is uncertain, and we often fear the unknown until we fully embrace the mystery that life is and learn to flow with it instead of resisting it.

12. Mindful Eating

A constantly distracted mind is an unhappy mind. Being present and more mindful is an experience of being alive more fully and joyful. Daily mindfulness practice has the potential to transform your life.

Slow down. Stop. Observe.

Mindfulness helps to create the physical time and the mental space to observe ourselves, our thoughts, and our tendencies.

It allows a more profound understanding, helping us change and evolve.

Do you ever find yourself eating without realising how much you've eaten or the taste of the food because you are doing something else? Being aware of your actions could be the key to understanding your behaviour, its consequences and implications, and therefore, changing your habits.

12.1. Mind full or mindful?

The main aspect of becoming healthier is probably in our minds.

Being mindless means the mind is somewhere else but not here on the present moment, while being mindful implies being fully present, paying attention to our experience as a neutral observer and without judgment of what's happening.

True health begins in the mind. We can join the gym, change our diet, or have some supplements as a starting point, but that alone is not enough in the long term.

If any of these actions are a reaction to compensate for a previous excess, to avoid some feelings or thoughts, or to distract from underlying issues, then we are making ourselves busy but not healthier.

Changing habits, reshaping behaviours, or having a different perspective on life start in our minds. True change always involves a shift in mindset and attitude.

Our overall well-being is the result of everything we do and what we choose not to do on a daily basis, and not what we do once a year or what we post on social media.

Being disconnected from the body can lead to ignoring its signals when it is full or hungry, or understanding what it needs, like driving a car blindly. And it can have consequences sooner or later that appear inexplicable, but often have roots in long-term lifestyle choices. In most cases, everything started much earlier, in a long slow process of choices through the years.

You can prevent those future consequences by bringing more awareness to your actions. This allows the mental space to see other options and consider different paths, therefore, creating a different history.

Mindless eating is when you are eating on autopilot without almost realising what you are putting inside your body. This might happen when you are watching TV while eating dinner, multitasking during lunch, busy with worries at breakfast, snacking on the go, or tired after a long day.

The key is to be mindful of your thoughts and actions at the moment you catch yourself losing attention. This can help you see where your feelings and habits are triggered and know yourself better. It will make you see your intentions and tendencies more clearly, allowing you to respond differently and create habits.

Make a pause
Slow down
Observe
Be present

12.2. What does it mean in practice?

Mindful eating means bringing awareness to the table. Here are some suggestions to help you with this and extend it to every part of your life, becoming more mindful and present in your daily activities.

Mindless eating

Most of the imbalances in eating, like binging or chocolate cravings, come from mindless eating, which mainly means thinking about something else while eating.

Do you ever find yourself losing track of what you're eating? Maybe you eat more when your mind is preoccupied with other things. If you notice this happening, try to slow down, stop, and observe it. You just need to start recognising these moments and bring your focus back to the present. It can help to focus on your breathing, ground yourself and feel your body sensations, or simply observe the details of your surroundings.

Slow down

Take a moment to slow down or stop and give yourself the mental space to reflect on your choices. Instead of rushing into things like taking extra portions or indulging in ice cream, question whether you truly need it and why you want it. Understanding your motivations will help you make wiser and new choices.

What can you notice?

What do you notice when you observe what's in your mind and pay attention to the present? Is it memories, worries, criticism, guiltiness, or excitement? Observe these thoughts with a certain detachment and realise how they are shaping your life experience.

Be grateful

Practicing gratitude can completely change your attitude and perception of a situation. Being thankful for the food and everyone involved in the food cycle process can transform how you perceive it. This gratitude can also help you be more mindful and make better choices as a result.

Be kind to yourself

Remember to talk kindly to yourself and use gentle words in your head. Judgmental words for yourself and others, resentment, perfectionism, blame, strict rules, guilt, or shame will just become your own jail sooner or later.

Food chain

Consider the entire food chain —where it comes from and everything that has to happen for you to get it.

The disconnection with this process may lead to forgetting where food is from and the true purpose of eating. The modern food environment and sedentary lifestyles may have a toll on our health and affect our eating habits. Understanding this chain can help change our relationship with food.

Cooking

Being involved in the process of buying and preparing your food can make you more in touch with what your meal is made of—a combination of ingredients with different properties, and not just food that you choose for its look, flavour, or price.

You can also use cooking as a meditative exercise or art, paying attention to the colours, smells, and textures. Have fun and be creative with it!

Body sensations

Remember to pay attention to the body and to the sensations from food, such as hunger, textures, flavours, aromas, and colours. Notice whether you feel stressed or calm. Eating too quickly can make it difficult to know when you're no longer hungry or when your body is satiated. Visualise your body as a collection of parts working together, each one with its own needs. By paying more attention to your body's signals and physical feelings, you can ground yourself in the present and be at home in your own skin.

13. Breath, Sunshine, Balance

Breathing techniques, getting regular sunshine, practicing activities for mind-body balance, dancing, and having meaningful connections with one another are also needed for the regulation of body functions, boosting the immune system, and as a source of energy and joy.

The quality of the breath determines the quality of your life.

The sun is necessary for life; most living beings depend on it to survive, and we are not different from the rest.

The mind-body connection is undeniable, and its balance and harmony are as much needed for our brain's health as everything else in life. Our motivation, mood states, sensitivity, empathy, attitude, thoughts, and inner peace are also essential to our overall health.

13.1. The quality of the breath

The quantity and quality of our breath impact the physical body, and just being mindful of it and bringing it to our awareness can benefit our health and calm down the nervous system.

Breathing

The science of breathing has been part of all traditional practices for centuries, telling us to mind and slow down our breath. Afterward, it has been demonstrated that our breathing affects the body and its chemical balance, and that there are scientific truths behind these traditional teachings of controlling the breath and paying attention to its quality. Nowadays, most modern studies and methods to improve physical and mental performance include breathing training exercises.

When we talk about the quality of breath, it may be a new concept for those who view breathing as only an automated process. However, how we inhale and exhale changes our body's physiology. It determines the amount of oxygen reaching all body cells and the pace of our heart. Oxygen is like fuel; the rate and delivery of it affect how our brain and muscles function.

The quality of our breath directly impacts the quality of our life. It is defined by its rate, rhythm, smoothness, regularity, and depth. The good news is that all these factors can be practiced and controlled—simply by starting paying attention to our breath and sometimes slowing it down.

Physical effects of deep breathing

What are the physical effects of regular deep breathing? Calming down the brain, regulating blood pressure, releasing stress on blood vessels, improving physical performance in sports, enhancing memory, and increasing the capacity to manage emotions. All these are benefits if we simply learn how to breathe and practice it regularly.

Most people take about 10 to 14 breaths per minute. However, slowing down to 6 breaths at a constant rhythm, keeping the same pace and smoothness, helps to relieve stress and focus.

For more examples, you can find enough literature and exercises on this topic, and the truth is that any of them can help you as long as you do them consistently and integrate them into your life.

13.2. Sunlight and balancing techniques

Sunlight, mind-body balancing techniques, and physical exercise are all needed for the brain's health, probably as much as the right food.

Singing and dancing

Singing, humming, and chanting can activate muscles and stimulate your vagus nerve, which is related to moods and mental well-being. Dancing, singing, and having fun make you feel good. In fact, they stimulate the physical parts of the brain related to feelings of joy—like a natural medicine!

Yoga, Tai Chi, and Kung Fu

All these disciplines have been proven to positively affect the physical chemistry responsible for harmony, the body's coordination and movements, the ability to cope with emotions, mind-body balance, and body awareness.

Sunshine

The sun is called the vitamin of happiness, and there are reasons for this. It's essential for the body to make vitamin D, which is related to moods. Symptoms of deficiency are sadness, demotivation, brain fog, and lethargy. The sun is like a source of joy and countries with less sunlight have higher rates of depression. Therefore, living outdoors can make troubles melt away and life look brighter under the sunshine.

Meditation and mindfulness

Meditation and mindfulness can change the brain, your life's perception, and the feelings underneath your actions. In other words, they can change the reality you live in. Enormous research over the last decades has proven their benefits scientifically, focusing on their effects on brain activity, the nervous system, and overall health.

In practice, such techniques can make us more aware of our thought processes and help to understand our emotions, providing tools to manage them. They can help us live more proactively instead of reactively and according to old habits.

14. Recapitulation

Good fats for the brain

Good fats are essential for the brain. As our brain is composed of 60 percent fat, it relies on healthy fats to build and repair its structure, and to function effectively. Deficiencies in good fats can be the underlying reasons for emotional imbalances, difficulty concentrating, mental fog, and early cognitive decline.

In the past, fat received a bad reputation due to the "low-fat products" trend, which were often high in sugars and actually contributed to weight gain. However, nowadays, this trend has already started to change.

The truth is the brain is hungry for good fats, so don't shy away from them. Find foods high in healthy fats that you like and create the habit to include them into your choices regularly.

Sugar and the brain

The brain is the organ that needs most glucose to function, which is the name for blood sugar, but its source is important. Natural sugars found in fruit, vegetables, and other unprocessed foods are packed with fibre and nutrients, serving as fuel for the brain's performance and well-being. However, excessive refined sugar consumption is unhealthy, leading to addictions, weight gain, fatigue, mood swings, type 2 diabetes, and other negative effects.

Check food labels, reduce ultra-processed sweets, choose more natural foods, and regulate your glucose. These changes can make your brain healthier and happier.

Gut and emotions

Our gut health and microbiota have a significant impact on our overall well-being, including our emotions and cognitive functions. There is a nervous system centralised in the belly that produces hormones and brain signals such as serotonin and dopamine, which is why it's often referred to as "the second brain." In addition to this, the health of the immune system is closely connected to our gut health, and also the digestion highly depends on it.

Issues in the gut can affect our whole body, including our mood, mental state, cognitive abilities, and immunity. Therefore, it's important to take a holistic approach, considering dietary choices, lifestyle factors, and emotional well-being. Our food choices, physical activity, stress levels, and sleep are all crucial factors in maintaining a healthy gut.

Vitamins for happiness

B vitamins play a role in many functions, especially energy production and brain performance. They are the keys to numerous reactions related to those processes, and the symptoms of their deficiency over long periods can be fatigue, tiredness, poor memory, low moods, depression, and general cognitive decline.

They are also essential for the immune system, skin health, and the brain and nervous system's development during pregnancy and childhood.

Food for emotional well-being

When we experience a feeling of excitement, joy, or sadness, it triggers reactions in the body, and different chemical substances are released. Can it also work the other way around? Can the release of some substances change the way we feel? Yes, it can.

Certain foods can affect these reactions and change the levels of chemicals, potentially causing some emotional or mood states. For instance, serotonin and dopamine are the messengers in conversations between neurons and play roles in motivation, pleasure, and connection. After doing exercise, our body releases components that boost our mood, while having a meal after being hungry can make us feel calmer and probably sleepy too.

You can help your body regulate these levels through dietary and lifestyle choices. Keep in mind that when your physical health is balanced, having a better attitude in life also becomes easier.

Not feeding worries

The body has its own ways of balancing itself without us needing to know how it works. So, it is okay if you didn't know it—your body has been handling it for you. We don't necessarily have to understand it, but now you do and can use it as an extra tool.

The overwhelming amount of mixed information about food and health might have also caused worry about problems that don't exist or created new ones. If you have concerns or fears, start by simply being aware of them and gradually modifying things that make you less healthy or limit your freedom. And remember that relaxation, joy, and fulfilment will also boost your health!

A holistic approach and consistency

A balanced diet and lifestyle maintained in the long term with consistency are essential for building up and preserving health. The things we do regularly have the greatest impact on our body, and not the exceptions. There are many foods and remedies with possible benefits for brain health, but they are most effective within a holistic approach over the long term.

Here are some general guidelines: include a variety of colourful fruits and vegetables, reduce your intake of ultra-processed food, ensure you get lean proteins and all nutrients from your diet, stay active, and get enough sleep. Incorporate fermented foods like yogurt, kefir, kombucha, or kimchi into your daily diet, balance your fat intake with more Omega 3 and unsaturated fats, and get enough B vitamins. Finally, remember to reduce stress and also prioritise joy, relaxation, fulfilment, and fun.

Breathing and sunshine

The science of breathing has been part of most medicinal traditions, emphasising to pay attention to the quality of our breath and its importance for health. Sunlight is also known to boost our moods and help the body's production of some essential vitamins for emotional well-being.

Considering all this, money can't be the excuse for not prioritising one's health. Engaging in simple activities such as deep breathing in fresh air, daily walks, enough sunlight exposure, and proper sleep continue to be some of the most effective remedies available today.

Ways to put all this into practice

Theory is silver, while practice is gold.

We can learn the theory, but actually realising its importance and putting it into practice is different. Otherwise, we may constantly perpetuate old tendencies or habits, become frustrated, build stories to justify ourselves, feel confused, see enemies everywhere, or doubt any new advice or information, always putting the blame outside of us. There is not a single method that works for all; many different lifestyles and dietary approaches can make you healthier if maintained consistently over the long term. And the truth is that your health doesn't only depend on your food and physical activity.

Your emotions, thoughts, fulfilment, relationships, and attitude in life also matter a great deal. Practices to observe your thought process, the associations in your memory, the assumptions you base your life on, your belief system, and understanding your predictability and tendencies can all be tools to navigate transitions, make conscious changes, move on, and evolve. Such approaches can be mindfulness, breathing, disciplines like yoga and tai chi, making art, taking a break from the routine, self-reflection, or simply being in silence more often. Those can help you pause and consider different perspectives, creating space and time for the new, like new thoughts, new associations of concepts, new meanings, and new patterns of behaviour in your beautiful mind.

Remember that everything takes time, so be patient with your process and persistent with your intention to evolve.

15. Smoothies & Salads

15.1.

Smoothies

Fruit

Use 2-3 different fruits. Add banana, avocado, or mango for a thicker consistency.

Liquid

Put water, yoghurt, and any type of unsweetened milk.

Nuts

Add one spoonful of nuts or nut butter. Peanuts give a strong flavour, chia seeds and flaxseeds make it more gelatinous, and roasted almonds give a sweet taste.

Spices and flavours

Flavour it with lemon, lime, mint, cinnamon, ginger, cocoa, vanilla, maca powder, matcha, or goji berries.

Veggies

Include some fresh spinach, kale, carrots, or celery.

Salads

Veggies

All veggies go well in salads, so use a variety of colours and types, making sure there are some leafy greens.

Protein

Fill up at least about a quarter of the plate with protein or a serving size of around 20-30 gr.

Nuts and dried fruit

Add 1-2 tbsp mixed nuts, seeds, and dried fruits for sweetness.

Sauce

Use the sauce to add extra healthy properties and not just flavour. You can make it with oils like flaxseeds, walnut, avocado, sesame, or olive oil, and condiments like fresh ginger, coriander, pepper, mint, and parsley.

Find more ideas on page 84.

Preparation

15.2 Brainy Smoothies

"Detox"

1 tbsp matcha
1 green apple
1 stalk celery
1/2 avocado
mint and lemon
water

"Wake up"

1/2 cup pineapple
1 green apple
1/2 celery stalk
1 cup spinach
fresh lemon or lime
water

"Aztecan"

1 cup soaked chia
seeds in yogurt
1 tsp cinnamon
2 tbsp cocoa
3 tbsp dates
3 tbsp any milk
Water

"Yummy"

3 tbsp almonds
2 tbsp cocoa
1 glass coconut milk
1 banana
2 tbsp dates
2 tbsp goji berries
1 tsp vanilla
water

"Tropical"

1/2 ripe mango
1 banana
2 tbsp pineapple
1 inch fresh ginger
fresh lemon/lime
water and ice mint

"Energy Boost"

1 tbsp cocoa and 2 tbsp raisins
1 banana and 1 cup coconut milk
2 tbsp walnuts and almonds
1 tbsp chia seeds soaked overnight
in the water or milk
water for a more liquid consistency

"Sweet dreams"

1 cup frozen berries
2 bananas
1 tbsp goji berries
3 tbsp yogurt or kefir
water

15.3. Joy Salads

Plants	Protein	Nuts & Fruits	Condiments
Starch-free	**Vegan**	**Seeds**	**Oils**
broccoli	beans	pumpkin	olive
spinach	chickpeas	sunflower	walnut
celery	hummus corn	chia	flaxseed
sprouts	pita	flax	avocado
asparagus	lentils	sesame	sesame
rocket	rice	poppy	coconut
lettuce	tofu	hemp	
kale	seitan		**Other**
cabbage	quinoa	**Nuts**	apple cider
artichoke	green peas		vinegar
zucchini	avocado	walnuts	lemon
cauliflower	edamame	almonds	pepper
tomatoes		hazelnuts	parsley
		brazil nuts	cilantro
	Non Vegan	peanuts	oregano
Starchy		pine	mint
	sardines		ginger
sweet	tuna		basil
potatoes	salmon	**Fruits**	mustard
potatoes	prawns	apples	honey
pumpkin	mussels	berries	pink salt
squash	eggs	goji berries	miso
taro	cheese	dried berries	yogurt
corn	chicken	raisins	
peas	ham	dates	
		mango	

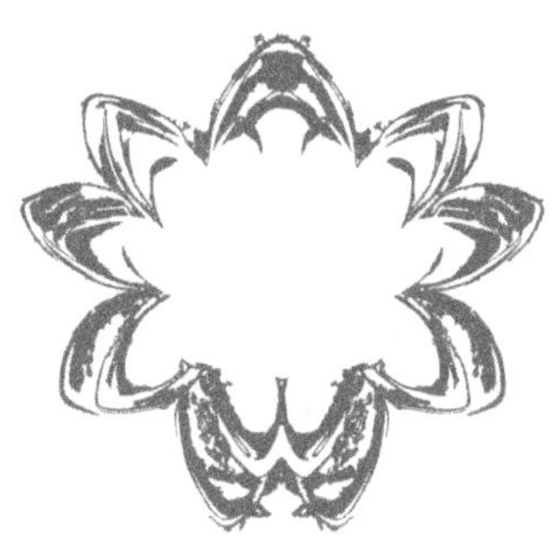

Mix and match from all columns

Include colours and a variety.

The more colours, variety, and food groups present, the richer in all nutrients your salad is.

Add spices, herbs, and good oils for taste.

Himalayan salt, pepper, rosemary, parsley, coriander, basil, mint, garlic, ginger, cumin, virgin olive oil, apple cider, or balsamic vinegar.

Wrap it up!

Use whole-grain, sourdough, or rye bread for a sandwich, or choose one of these creative gluten-free options: Lettuce leaves as a veggie version, rice paper as a Vietnamese-style roll, or nori seaweed as a Japanese style.

Last Thoughts

Now, digest it...

You have just been reading lots of information that may have made you think or question things.

Now it's time to digest it all.

Let it rest and allow the information to settle in your mind, come back to revisit it from time to time to slowly integrate it into your set of knowledge, and make it part of your daily habits and routine.

That is the main point of it; to eventually apply it and improve your quality of life. After all, theory without application can just be frustrating, right?

You can use the guidelines and lists throughout this book as reminders, helping you make gradual improvement little by little every day, creating almost effortlessly new long-term habits.

Also, mind your happiness and peace of mind.

You have likely heard enough contradictory information, names of conditions that probably don't apply to you, and problems that are not yours to solve. The modern hyperconnected world can be too overwhelming and our minds are not designed to deal with all opinions, problems, and conflicts all at once.

It might be time to release those overwhelming feelings and worries instead of adding more to them, while practicing tolerance, patience, and forgiveness. Finding more joy and peace in your life will surely contribute to your overall wellbeing. Health is about balance and is simpler than what the health industry has led us to believe. If it feels too complicated, strict, or expensive, you most likely need to revise your approach.

Finally, remain open to learning and evolving.

"Change" means much more than just doing something differently; it involves challenging assumptions, concepts, and ideas. It is related to the constant movement and ongoing flow inherent in life. Give yourself time and see this book just as a small step in your journey along the never-ending path of learning.

Food Wisdom Series

Food Wisdom is a series of practical short guides for learning about holistic health and nutrition in simple and accessible ways. These are other titles in the series:

The 10-Day Energy & Habits Challenge

A 10-day plan to learn how to raise and maintain energy levels and to integrate wholesome and healthy long-term habits. You will get the principles to apply, a set of menus and examples, options to adapt it to the most common diets nowadays, and tools to put all this into practice.

Become Your Own Food Master

Become your own guide in modern times and a master of your health. Learn the fundamentals of nutrition, understand your body and its principles, and how to make the best choices for your holistic well-being.

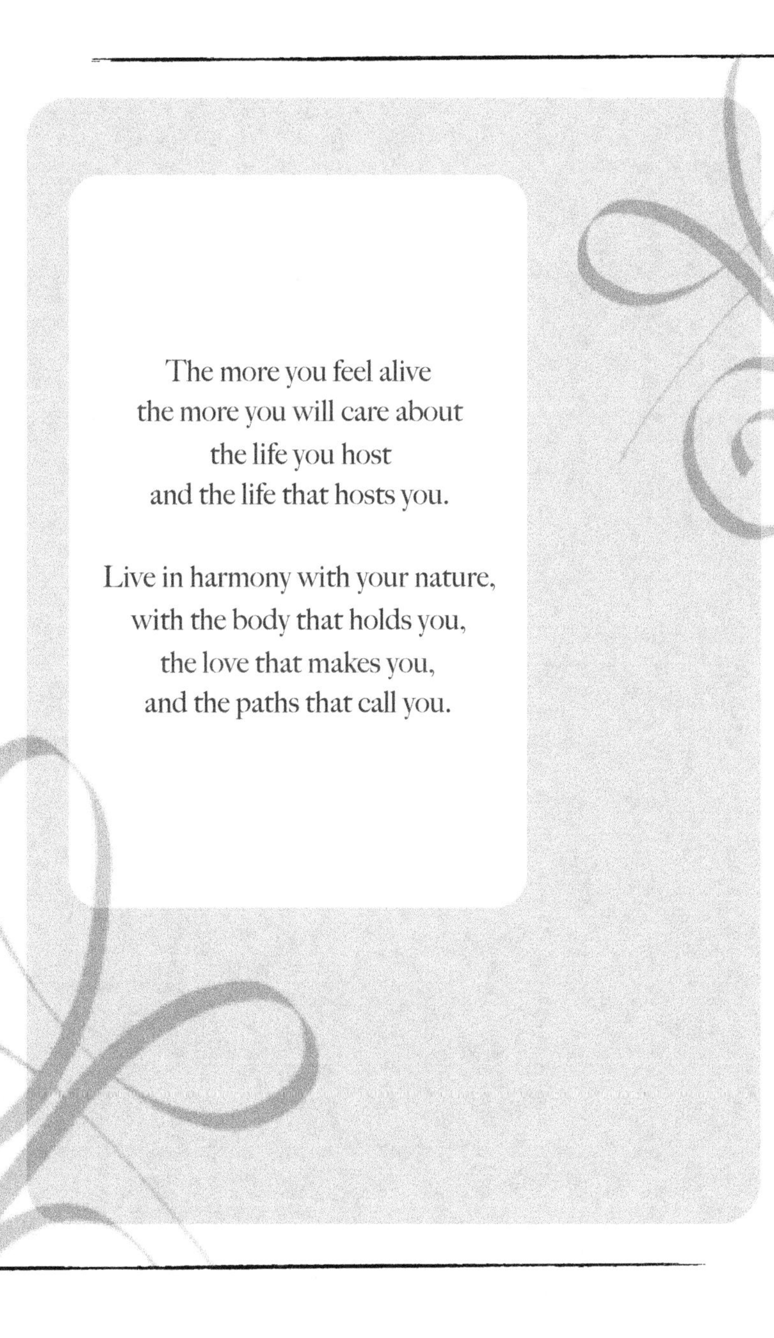

The more you feel alive
the more you will care about
the life you host
and the life that hosts you.

Live in harmony with your nature,
with the body that holds you,
the love that makes you,
and the paths that call you.